CELIAC DISEASE DIET COOKBOOK

Gluten-Free Recipes For Optimal Digestive Health: Easy, Delicious, And Nutritious Meals For Managing Immune System And Enhancing Well-Being

DR. AMARI VALERIE

TABLE OF CONTENTS

BONUS:

7 days meal plan recipes, ingredients, and detailed preparatory guidelines for Celiac Disease

7 Desserts procedural recipes for Celiac Disease and guidelines

7 Smoothies procedural recipes for Celiac Disease and guidelines

DISCLAIMER

The information provided in this book, is for educational and informational purposes only and is not intended as medical advice. The content is not a substitute for professional medical advice, diagnosis, or treatment. Always seek the advice of your physician or other qualified health provider with any questions you may have regarding a medical condition. Never disregard professional medical advice or delay in seeking it because of something you have read in this book.

The dietary suggestions and recipes in this book are based on general guidelines and may not be suitable for everyone. Individual responses to foods can vary, and it is important to consult with a healthcare professional before making any significant changes to your diet.

The author and publisher of this book do not claim to cure or treat any medical condition. The information provided is based on research and personal experience and is intended to help readers make informed decisions about their diet and health.

Furthermore, I the author do not endorse any specific products, brands, treatments, or services that may be mentioned in this book. Any references to products, services, websites, or organizations are provided for informational purposes only and do not constitute an endorsement or recommendation by the author. The inclusion of such references does not imply any association, sponsorship, or affiliation between the author and the referenced entities.

The recipes and dietary suggestions in this book are designed to be safe and healthful. However, readers should use their own discretion and consult with a healthcare professional when necessary, especially if they have allergies, sensitivities, or other dietary restrictions.

By using this book, you acknowledge and agree that the author and publisher shall not be held liable for any loss or damage, including but not limited to special, incidental, consequential, or other damages, resulting from the use of the information and recipes contained in this book.

ABOUT THIS BOOK

This "Celiac Disease Diet Cookbook" is an essential resource for individuals who are navigating the complications of celiac disease and transitioning to a gluten-free diet. Beginning with an exhaustive introduction that provides a comprehensive account of celiac disease, including its symptoms and description, this book delves into the critical role of a gluten-free diet in the management of this autoimmune condition. It underscores the severe long-term health repercussions of untreated celiac disease and offers crucial resources for further reading and support, guaranteeing that readers are adequately informed and encouraged throughout their journey.

The primary emphasis of this book is on the fundamentals of a gluten-free diet, which include the identification of gluten, its typical location, and the foods you should stay away from. It encompasses practical advice on identifying concealed gluten sources by perusing labels, as well as suggestions for dining out and socializing. The incorporation of gluten-free alternatives facilitates readers' uncomplicated adaptation and avoids any sense of deprivation, while simultaneously increasing their awareness of the gluten-free lifestyle.

The benefits of a gluten-free lifestyle are underscored, with an in-depth examination of the enhancements in digestive health, immune system function, energy levels, and mental lucidity that numerous individuals have reported. This book emphasizes the long-term health benefits of a gluten-free diet, offering a compelling rationale for adhering to it beyond the temporary relief of acute symptoms.

Comprehensive recommendations are provided for the establishment of a gluten-free kitchen, including the following safe culinary procedures, the prevention of cross-contamination, and the provisioning of a gluten-free larder. The guidance provided on gluten-free culinary equipment and meal planning enables readers to establish a secure and efficient kitchen environment, thereby enabling them to prepare meals with assurance and safety.

Common questions and concerns are addressed, including the methods for managing inadvertent gluten exposure, preventing nutritional deficiencies, and adhering to a gluten-free diet on a budget. This book also addresses social issues, providing readers with practical information on how to navigate social situations and ensure that they are well-prepared to live gluten-free in all aspects of their lives.

This cookbook seamlessly transitions into practical application, with chapters that are specifically designed for various meal times and circumstances. This book encompasses a wide range of dishes to accommodate a diverse array of preferences and dietary needs, from breakfast to supper, nibbles to desserts. Each recipe segment, including breakfast, lunch, and supper, features delectable, straightforward recipes that illustrate the versatility and enjoyment of gluten-free cookery.

Special occasion recipes enable readers to celebrate holidays and anniversaries without compromising their nutritional needs. This book also offers long-term strategies for maintaining a gluten-free diet, underscoring the importance of maintaining motivation and establishing a supportive community. This comprehensive book concludes with recommendations for dining out and traveling, guaranteeing that readers can confidently maintain their gluten-free lifestyle, irrespective of their location.

In general, this "Celiac Disease Diet Cookbook" is not merely a compilation of recipes; it is a comprehensive guide to leading a healthy, fulfilling gluten-free lifestyle. It offers readers the necessary knowledge, skills, and motivation to effectively manage their celiac disease and maximize the benefits of a gluten-free diet.

CHAPTER ONE

Introduction

Celiac disease is an autoimmune disorder in which the small intestinal lining is destroyed by an immune response that is triggered by the consumption of gluten, a protein found in wheat, barley, and rye. This injury can result in a variety of health concerns and reduces the absorption of nutrition. Blood testing for specific antibodies and a biopsy of the small intestine are employed to diagnose celiac disease and corroborate intestinal injury.

Diagnosis And Symptoms

Symptoms of celiac disease may include diarrhea, bloating, and gastrointestinal discomfort, as well as anemia, lethargy, and skin lesions. Antibodies, including anti-tissue transglutaminase (tTG) and endomysial antibodies (EMA), are frequently detected through serological assays. An endoscopic biopsy is frequently conducted in response to a positive result to detect villous atrophy in the small intestine.

The Significance Of Gluten-Free Diets

The only effective treatment for celiac disease is a strict gluten-free diet. The removal of gluten facilitates the regeneration of the small intestine, alleviates symptoms, and prevents further injury. This involves refraining from consuming any meals or products that contain wheat, barley, or rye, including less obvious sources such as certain condiments and processed foods.

Attentive label reading and awareness of cross-contamination concerns are essential strategies for managing the condition.

Uncontrolled Celiac Disease's Long-Term Health Consequences

Celiac disease can result in severe long-term health complications, including osteoporosis, infertility, neurological disorders, and an elevated risk of certain malignancies, including intestinal lymphoma if left untreated. In addition to alleviating acute symptoms, adhering to a gluten-free diet significantly reduces long-term health concerns, thereby improving one's overall quality of life.

Additional Reading And Support Resources

Individuals who have recently been diagnosed with celiac disease or need additional support have access to a variety of resources. The Celiac Disease Foundation and the National Celiac Association are among the websites that offer a wealth of information, recipes, and community support. Books such as "Gluten Is My Bitch" and "The Gluten-Free Bible" provide both entertainment and practical advice. Additionally, participating in local support organizations can facilitate the exchange of ideas and experiences.

The Basics Of A Gluten-Free Diet

A gluten-free diet is characterized by the elimination of all foods that contain gluten, a protein that is present in wheat, barley, and rye. This entails refraining from consuming the majority of bread, pasta, cereals, and processed dishes that contain these carbohydrates. All of the following are considered safe: fresh fruits, vegetables, livestock, seafood, beans, legumes, nuts, and gluten-free cereals like rice, quinoa, and maize. Rice or quinoa pasta, gluten-free breads, and gluten-free flour treats are all acceptable alternatives. It is imperative to meticulously read labels and acquire the ability to identify concealed gluten in foods, including malt, soy sauce, and specific thickeners. To manage dining out, it is possible to select establishments that offer gluten-free options, inform the staff of dietary restrictions, and prevent cross-contamination. It may be necessary to carry your gluten-free dishes to ensure safe dining in social situations.

What Is Gluten And Where Can It Be Found?

Wheat, barley, and rye are sources of the protein gluten. It contributes to the preservation of the shape of meals by providing elasticity and moisture. Cereals, bread, pasta, baked goods, and a variety of processed dishes all contain gluten. Gluten is also present in certain medications and supplements, as well as in condiments, stews, and dressings, as a thickening agent. These sources must be completely avoided by individuals with celiac disease to prevent adverse health effects.

Foods That Should Be Avoided

Individuals with celiac disease are required to refrain from consuming any products that contain wheat, barley, rye, or derivatives. This consists of rye bread, barley malt, and wheat flour. Gluten may be utilized as a thickener or flavor enhancer in numerous processed foods, including sauces, stews, and munchies. Other typical sources include beer, malted beverages, and certain desserts. To reduce the risk of cross-contamination, it is crucial to cook items in a gluten-free environment.

Alternatives That Are Devoid Of Gluten

A variety of gluten-free alternatives are available to substitute for gluten-containing meals. Almond flour, rice flour, and coconut flour are gluten-free flour that can be employed in cookery. Gluten-free pastas are easily accessible and are typically produced from rice, quinoa, or maize. Delectable alternatives are offered by gluten-free bread and treats that are made from cereals such as buckwheat, sorghum, and millet. Additionally, numerous establishments offer gluten-free alternatives to conventional items such as cereals, biscuits, and crackers, thereby simplifying the process of maintaining a varied and satisfying diet.

Reading Food Labels And Detecting Hidden Gluten

It is imperative to read food labels with care to prevent the consumption of gluten. Important ingredients to consider include malt, brewer's yeast, wheat, barley, and rye. Some products may not explicitly mention gluten; however, they do contain it in additives like hydrolyzed vegetable protein or modified dietary starch. While certified gluten-free labeling can provide assurance, it is crucial to exercise caution. It is crucial to inspect condiments, dressings, and seasonings for concealed gluten. Oats should not be used unless they are designated as gluten-free, as they are susceptible to cross-contamination during the manufacturing process.

Some Advice For Dining And Social Events

Select restaurants that offer gluten-free menus or inform the staff of your dietary restrictions to ensure that they understand the importance of preventing cross-contamination when dining out. Conducting menu research can assist you in identifying secure alternatives. You may prevent gluten-related accidents by bringing your gluten-free cuisine to social gatherings. To guarantee your safety, be forthright with your hosts, and do not hesitate to inquire about the ingredients and preparation methods.

CHAPTER TWO

Benefits Of A Gluten-Free Lifestyle

Enhanced Digestive Function

Intestinal health can be significantly enhanced for celiac patients by transitioning to a gluten-free diet. Eliminating gluten, which is found in wheat, barley, and rye, can alleviate symptoms such as constipation, diarrhea, bloating, and flatulence. For instance, substituting conventional pasta with rice or quinoa pasta may alleviate digestive problems.

Consuming a greater variety of naturally gluten-free meals, including fruits, vegetables, lean proteins, and dairy products, can also contribute to the enhancement of one's digestive health.

Enhanced Immune System Function

By reducing inflammation and facilitating the gut's recovery, a gluten-free diet can enhance the immune system's functionality. When celiac patients consume gluten, their immune system incorrectly targets the small intestine, resulting in inadequate nutritional absorption and injury. The immune system can function more efficiently without being compromised by abstaining from gluten. Consuming foods that are abundant in vitamins and minerals, such as almonds, seeds, and verdant vegetables, can enhance one's immune system.

Enhanced Vitality Levels

It is common for individuals with celiac disease to experience chronic fatigue as a consequence of nutritional deficiencies that are caused by intestinal injury. A gluten-free diet can aid in the restoration of the intestines and the improvement of nutritional assimilation, which can lead to increased energy levels. For instance, beginning the day with a gluten-free oatmeal dish that is garnished with almonds and fresh berries may provide you with the energy you need to get through the morning. A diet that is well-balanced and contains a sufficient amount of protein, healthful lipids, and carbohydrates is necessary to sustain high energy levels.

Improvement In Mood And Mental Clarity

Brain clarity and emotional improvement may be facilitated by a gluten-free diet. The avoidance of gluten can alleviate the symptoms of "brain fog" and mood fluctuations that are frequently reported by celiac disease patients. Brain function can be enhanced by consuming foods that are rich in omega-3 fatty acids, such as salmon and flaxseeds, as well as antioxidant-rich fruits and vegetables. Cognitive performance and emotional well-being can be enhanced by maintaining hydration and adhering to a nutritious diet.

Adopting a gluten-free diet has long-term health benefits by preventing the consequences of untreated celiac disease, including osteoporosis, infertility, and certain malignancies. Individuals who adhere to a strict gluten-free diet can reduce their risk of developing significant health issues by maintaining the health and functionality of their intestines. Consuming a variety of gluten-free whole grains, including buckwheat, millet, and brown rice, in addition to a varied diet of fruits and vegetables, will help to preserve overall health and avert potential health issues.

CHAPTER THREE

Establishing A Gluten-Free Kitchen

To ensure that your kitchen is gluten-free, it is important to thoroughly clean all surfaces and replace any porous equipment, such as wooden utensils or cutting boards, that may contain gluten.

Ensure that any shared appliances, such as colanders and toasters, are either gluten-free or have distinct variants for gluten-containing items. To prevent unintentional contamination, it is important to use containers that are properly labeled and to position gluten-free foods at the top of the shelf. By designating a separate workstation for the preparation of gluten-free meals, the likelihood of cross-contamination is diminished, thereby ensuring that the kitchen is a secure environment for Celiac patients.

Must-Have Gluten-Free Pantry Items

Gluten-free flour (such as rice, almond, and coconut flour), gluten-free pasta, and certified gluten-free cereals are essential components of a gluten-free pantry. Incorporate natural gluten-free cereals, such as buckwheat, millet, and quinoa. Ensure that your pantry is stocked with a variety of gluten-free culinary ingredients, including baking powder and xanthan gum. Additionally, it is advisable to maintain a diverse selection of gluten-free condiments, sauces, and munchies to facilitate meal preparation and prevent inadvertent gluten ingestion.

Tips For Preventing Cross-Contaminations:

In a gluten-free kitchen, it is imperative to prevent cross-contamination. Separate cutting boards, utensils, and apparatus should be employed when preparing with gluten-free ingredients. Containers and storage locations must be plainly labeled as gluten-free. To eliminate any gluten residue, it is important to regularly clean culinary surfaces and counters. To prevent contact with gluten, prepare gluten-free foods first or use alternative timings and locations when cooking. Simple yet beneficial precautions include washing one's hands and changing mittens when handling gluten and gluten-free meals.

Best Practices For Cooking Safely

Set up a system of meticulous cleansing and organized stowage to guarantee the safety of the kitchen. Store gluten-free products in containers that are sealed and have easily readable labels. It is advisable to refrain from using shared condiments, as they may be contaminated with gluten-containing food particles. Specialist sponges and dishcloths should be employed to clean gluten-free dishes. Ensure that the kitchen is a safe environment for gluten-free cookery by regularly sterilizing kitchen surfaces and equipment and educating all family members on the importance of adhering to these measures.

Gadgets And Tools For Gluten-Free Cooking

Having the appropriate kitchen equipment may facilitate the process of preparing gluten-free meals. Purchase a high-quality gluten-free breadmaker, a distinct toaster, and nonstick cookware. Line baking vessels with parchment paper or silicone baking mats to prevent them from adhering.

A digital kitchen scale can assist in the accurate measurement of gluten-free flour. A spiralizer is another useful instrument for generating gluten-free vegetable noodles, which add variety to your dishes. Additionally, a food processor is used to create gluten-free flour and dough.

Tips For Meal Planning And Preparation

Efficient meal planning and preparation are essential for maintaining a gluten-free diet. Make sure you have all the necessary gluten-free products by creating purchasing lists and planning your meals. Batch preparing and freezing portions can provide convenient, secure meal options throughout the week, as well as save time.

To guarantee appropriate nutrition, it is crucial to include a diverse selection of protein sources, vegetables, and gluten-free cereals in your meal planning. Separate and store foods in meal prep containers to prevent cross-contamination and maintain an organized kitchen.

CHAPTER FOUR

Managing Accidental Gluten Exposure

Remaining vigilant for cross-contamination and comprehending the appropriate course of action in the event of accidental gluten exposure are essential components of managing it. If you suspect that you have consumed gluten, it is important to maintain hydration and consume activated charcoal to aid in its binding to your stomach. Rest as much as possible and adhere to a bland diet consisting of rice, bananas, and chicken bouillon for the next 24 hours.

Maintain a record of your symptoms to provide your physician with personalized recommendations, and ensure that you always have gluten-digesting enzyme capsules on hand as a precaution.

The Prevention Of Nutritional Deficiencies

To prevent the nutritional deficiencies that are linked to celiac disease, ensure that your diet includes a variety of naturally gluten-free foods that are rich in essential nutrients. oily fish such as salmon and fortified gluten-free cereals are all excellent sources of iron and fiber, as are leafy vegetables, nuts, seeds, and legumes. Consult with a nutritionist to regularly evaluate your nutritional status and adjust your diet or supplements as necessary. Additionally, consider taking a daily multivitamin that is specifically intended for celiac patients.

Gluten-Free On A Budget

Eating gluten-free on a budget can be achieved by focusing on complete, naturally gluten-free foods, such as rice, potatoes, legumes, and seasonal fruits and vegetables. Purchase these ingredients in abundance, prepare meals at home, and refrain from purchasing expensive gluten-free packaged products. Utilize applications and websites that offer gluten-free coupons and discounts, and organize your meals to reduce waste. Additionally, participating in a local gluten-free support group can guide the most cost-effective methods of purchasing and preparing meals.

Social Challenges And Strategies For Overcoming Them

Social interactions with celiac disease can be challenging to manage, but it is crucial to plan. When dining out, seek out restaurants that provide gluten-free menus and contact them in advance to discuss your preferences. Please bring a gluten-free dish to share and inform the host of your dietary restrictions. Connecting with other celiac patients can provide moral support and shared techniques while practicing courteous but firm communication about your dietary requirements can help you avoid awkward situations.

Frequently Asked Questions Regarding Gluten-Free Living

There are numerous challenges associated with living gluten-free, including the permissibility of consuming grains (provided that they are labeled as gluten-free) and the management of medication. It is essential to closely read food labels and be aware of potential gluten sources, such as sauces and processed dishes. These issues can be addressed and continuous support can be provided by the following: regular consultations with a healthcare physician, membership in support groups, and ongoing education through reputable celiac organizations.

CHAPTER FIVE

Comprehending Gluten And Its Origins

Gluten, a protein, is present in wheat, barley, rye, and their derivatives. In individuals with celiac disease, the small intestine can be destroyed by an immunological reaction that is induced by the consumption of gluten. Ensure that food labels are thoroughly examined to prevent the presence of gluten.

Bread, pasta, cereals, and numerous processed dishes are frequently contaminated with gluten. Sauces and condiments, as well as certain medications and supplements, contain concealed sources. While purchasing, seek out "gluten-free" labels or certified gluten-free symbols.

The Fundamentals Of A Gluten-Free Diet

Fruits, vegetables, meat, fish, eggs, nuts, seeds, and lentils are all inherently gluten-free foods that can be consumed on a gluten-free diet. Rice, maize, quinoa, and potatoes are all regarded as safe cereals and starches. Cross-contamination is a potential hazard; therefore, it is imperative to utilize distinct culinary equipment and prepare meals in a sanitary environment. Checking for gluten-free certification regularly can help ensure that the product is safe for consumption.

Adopting A Gluten-Free Diet

Transitioning to a gluten-free diet requires more than just modifying one's diet; it also requires a modification to one's daily regimen. To begin, substitute gluten-free alternatives for staples such as traditional bread. Plan your meals and investigate gluten-free options to ensure that your diet remains engaging and enjoyable.

To prevent gluten exposure at social events and meals out, inform your family and acquaintances about your dietary needs.

Common Errors To Avoid

A common misconception is that all gluten-free meals are nutritious; however, numerous processed gluten-free products are high in sugar and cholesterol. Another error is the failure to read labels accurately, which may lead to the accidental ingestion of gluten. Cross-contamination in the kitchen is another prevalent issue; it is recommended to use distinct toasters, cutting boards, and utensils for gluten-free dishes. Additionally, it is important to be cautious of the bulk containers at supermarkets, as they can rapidly become contaminated with gluten from other products.

Practical Advice For Novices

Sticking to full, unadulterated foods and progressively incorporating gluten-free equivalents may be beneficial for individuals who are new to a gluten-free diet. Participate in online forums or support groups to exchange experiences and obtain advice. It may be challenging to dine out, so it is advisable to conduct a thorough search for gluten-free restaurants and communicate your needs directly with the staff. Maintain a food journal to track your reactions to various meals and adjust your diet accordingly. Resources and applications, including the Gluten-Free Allergy-Free Marketplace of the Celiac Disease Foundation, may prove advantageous in your pursuit.

CHAPTER SIX

Breakfast Recipes

Avocado toast on gluten-free bread, yogurt parfaits with gluten-free granola and fresh cherries, and overnight oats prepared with gluten-free oats and almond milk are all simple and quick gluten-free breakfast ideas. These dishes are effortless to prepare and are perfect for a rushed morning, as they contain a well-balanced ratio of fiber, healthy lipids, and protein.

Blend a banana, berries, and almond milk with verdant greens such as spinach or kale to create a nutritious smoothie. For an additional nutritional boost, incorporate a scoop of gluten-free protein powder or chia seeds. These beverages are quick to prepare and can be tailored to accommodate your nutritional needs and flavor preferences.

Gluten-Free Pancakes and Waffles: Utilize a gluten-free flour blend to prepare delectable gluten-free pancakes and waffles. Combine flour, eggs, milk (or a dairy-free substitute), baking powder, and a small amount of salt to make pancakes. Achieve a crispier texture by incorporating a small amount of additional fat, such as heated butter or coconut oil, into a mixture similar to that used for waffles. Incorporate fresh fruit and pure maple syrup to create a delectable breakfast delight.

Creative Egg-Based Dishes Enhance your morning with innovative egg-based dishes, such as a gluten-free quiche with an almond flour crust or a frittata that is filled with vegetables. Prepare a gluten-free burrito with scrambled eggs, black beans, avocado, and salsa for a speedy breakfast, or scramble eggs with spinach, tomatoes, and cheese.

Almond flour, coconut flour, or a combination of gluten-free flour can be employed to produce delectable muffins and breads. Banana bread, blueberry pastries, and zucchini bread are among the most popular choices. Utilize xanthan gum and gluten-free baking powder to facilitate the dough's expansion and attain the desired texture. These baked goods can be prepared in advance and stored for a quick and enjoyable breakfast.

Lunch Recipes

Salads That Are Both Delicious And Gluten-Free

Selecting fresh ingredients and combining them in a manner that is both healthful and palatable is the process of preparing a gluten-free salad. Start with a base of verdant greens, such as kale or spinach. Incorporate a diverse array of vibrant vegetables, such as cucumbers, bell peppers, and cherry tomatoes. Chickpeas, hard-boiled eggs, or grilled chicken are all excellent protein sources. Top with a straightforward vinaigrette consisting of honey, lemon juice, and olive oil. For an additional burst of texture and nutrient content, incorporate almonds or seeds. For instance, a gluten-free, substantial, and delectable option is a quinoa and black bean salad with avocado.

Hearty Soups And Stews

Soups and stews may serve as a gratifying and substantial lunchtime option. Commence with a gluten-free bouillon, such as chicken, beef, or vegetable. Includes a diverse array of vegetables, including celery, carrots, and potatoes. Protein can be supplemented with beans, lentils, or meat fragments. Thyme, rosemary, and bay leaves are among the spices and herbs that enhance the flavor. For a warm gluten-free supper, a beef and vegetable stew that has been prepared to perfection is a fantastic example. The stew is made with soft pieces of meat, root vegetables, and a rich broth.

Sandwiches And Wraps That Are Devoid Of Gluten

Sandwiches and wraps that are gluten-free may be equally as delicious as their conventional counterparts. Utilize gluten-free tortillas or bread as a foundation. Load them with lean proteins, including turkey, prosciutto, and grilled vegetables. Incorporate fresh vegetables, such as cucumbers, tomatoes, and lettuce, to provide a satisfying texture. Distribute gluten-free condiments, such as mayonnaise or mustard. A turkey and avocado sandwich is a common example of a convenient and satisfying meal option. It is made by combining a gluten-free tortilla, sliced turkey breast, avocado, lettuce, and a small amount of mustard.

Lunch Containers That Are Both Nutritious And Effortless

supper containers are a straightforward and adaptable method of preparing a nourishing gluten-free supper. Start with a base, such as blended greens, quinoa, or brown rice. In addition to vegetables such as roasted sweet potatoes, broccoli, and cherry tomatoes, toppings may consist of boiled eggs, tofu, or broiled poultry. Apply a straightforward condiment or vinaigrette. For instance, a nutrient-dense and delicious meal can be achieved by combining grilled chicken, roasted vegetables, and tahini vinaigrette in a quinoa bowl.

Ideas For A Quick Lunch On Busy Days.

It is imperative to prepare for those chaotic days when you require a quick meal. Rice cakes, nut butter, and pre-washed salad greens are all essential gluten-free items that should be included in your pantry. Simple dishes, such as a rice cake with avocado and baby carrots or a fast salad with pre-cooked chicken, mixed vegetables, and a light vinaigrette, can be prepared in a matter of minutes. A lunch option that is both nutritious and delicious is a Greek yogurt parfait topped with fresh cherries and gluten-free granola. It is a fast and effortless meal.

Dinner Recipes

Delectable gluten-free main dishes: The process of creating delectable gluten-free main dishes is both simple and enjoyable. Indulge in herb-roasted chicken that has been marinated in olive oil, garlic, thyme, and rosemary, and is served alongside roasted vegetables. An additional exceptional alternative is a bell pepper that has been stuffed with quinoa, black beans, maize, and seasonings like chili powder and cumin. Enhance the flavor of your entrée while maintaining its safety and flavor by incorporating gluten-free broth and seasonings.

Nutritious, gluten-free side dishes: Serve gluten-free side dishes that are nutritious in conjunction with your primary meals. A refreshing, astringent cucumber and tomato salad that is prepared with fresh dill, lemon juice, and olive oil may be a welcome addition. Conversely, consider a sweet potato mash that is rich in nutrients, made with coconut milk and a sprinkle of cinnamon. Both options are effortless to prepare and offer a nutritious assortment of dishes.

Comfort foods that have been rendered gluten-free: It is entirely practicable to consume comfort foods while adhering to a gluten-free diet. Make a comforting dish by combining gluten-free macaroni with a buttery sauce made from cheddar cheese, milk, and gluten-free flour. Another recipe that is highly regarded is a substantial gluten-free meatloaf that is prepared using gluten-free breadcrumbs, minced beef, shallots, and seasonings. The meatloaf is then cooked to perfection.

Your culinary horizons can be expanded by consuming gluten-free dishes from other countries. Coconut milk, green curry paste, chicken, and additional vegetables, including snap peas and bell peppers, are the components of Thai chicken curry, a dish that is both uncomplicated and delicious. For a complete meal, serve it with jasmine rice. For a taste of Italy, consider gluten-free spaghetti primavera, which is made by tossing gluten-free pasta in a light olive oil and garlic sauce and blending it with seasonally fresh vegetables.

Effective meal planning and preparation are indispensable for adhering to a gluten-free diet. Begin by devising a weekly meal plan that incorporates a variety of cereals, vegetables, and proteins. Batch cookery may be advantageous; for instance, one may prepare a substantial quantity of gluten-free chili to consume over the course of several days. Ensure that all products are gluten-free by inspecting the labels and maintaining a clean kitchen to prevent cross-contamination.

CHAPTER SEVEN

Appetizers And Snacks

Rice cakes topped with avocado and cherry tomatoes, yogurt with fresh fruits and honey, and cucumber segments with hummus are all quick and simple gluten-free snack options. These options are not only gluten-free, but they are also rich in nutrients that will provide you with energy throughout the day.

Bacon-wrapped dates, toasted gluten-free bread with tomatoes and basil, and small caprese skewers with cherry tomatoes, mozzarella balls, and fresh basil leaves are all simple appetizers that are perfect for gatherings. All of your guests will be taken aback by the bite-sized delights.

Prepare gluten free snacks and dips at home by utilizing sweet potatoes or maize tortillas. Serve them with guacamole, salsa, or a creamy spinach artichoke mixture after slicing them thinly and baking until golden. This combination produces a refreshment that is both nutritious and enjoyable.

Mix gluten-free oats, almonds, dried fruits, and a binding agent like peanut butter or honey to produce your nutritious snack bars. Press the mixture into a pan, refrigerate until it is firm, and then cut it into bars. Energy spheres, which are formed by combining dates, almonds, and cocoa powder and cooling them, are an option for bite-sized treats.

Gluten-free pretzels, homemade popcorn, apple segments with almond butter, and cheese sticks are all kid-friendly gluten-free treats. Additionally, you may utilize a variety of fresh fruits to create vibrant and colorful fruit kabobs that are both nutritious and appealing to children.

Delectable Gluten-Free Cakes And Cookies

Almond flour, coconut flour, or a combination of rice flour and tapioca starch is used to create gluten-free cakes and pastries, which are created by substituting traditional wheat flour with alternatives. Begin by adhering to a dependable gluten-free recipe and accurately measuring the ingredients. Utilize guar gum or xanthan gum to replicate the pliability of gluten. Vanilla sponge pastries and gluten-free chocolate chip biscuits are among the most popular options. To prevent adhering, it is essential to preheat your oven and use parchment paper. Ensure that all ingredients, including the baking powder, are gluten-free.

Homemade Gluten-Free Pies And Tarts

To prepare gluten-free pies and tarts, begin by preparing a pastry that is a blend of gluten-free flour, including sorghum flour, potato starch, and tapioca flour, as well as butter or a dairy-free substitute. Roll the dough between two sheets of parchment paper to prevent it from adhering. Fill your crust with fresh fruit, custard, or chocolate ganache, ensuring that all ingredients are gluten-free. To maintain the form and texture of the dish, bake it according to the recipe instructions and allow it to chill before dividing.

Dessert Alternatives That Are Devoid Of Dairy And Gluten

It may be challenging, but it can also be rewarding, to combine dairy-free and gluten-free alternatives. Substitute plant-based milk (such as almond, coconut, or soy) and lipids (such as coconut oil or margarine) in your recipes. Develop a chocolate mousse that is both dairy-free and gluten-free by incorporating avocado, cocoa powder, and a natural sweetener like maple syrup. Alternatively, prepare fruit-based desserts, such as baked pears stuffed with almonds and candied fruits or sorbets. Read the labels for gluten and dairy components at all times.

Suggestions For Baking Gluten-Free

To achieve success in gluten-free cookery, certain modifications are necessary. Initially, it is imperative to employ a gluten-free flour blend that is of superior quality and has been specifically formulated for baking. Binding agents, such as xanthan gum or psyllium fiber, are employed to replicate the texture of gluten. Ensure that your measurements are precise; the result may be considerably impacted by an excessive or insufficient amount.

Ensure that your oven is thoroughly preheated and that an oven thermometer is employed to guarantee precision. It is advisable to allow baked goods to chill completely before slicing them, as they may be more fragile than their gluten-free counterparts.

Nutritious Sweets

To create healthy gluten-free delectable treats, opt for natural sweeteners such as honey, maple syrup, or dates in place of processed sugars. Supplement your diet with nutrient-dense items, including preserved fruits, seeds, and almonds. Energy balls, which are composed of dates, almonds, cocoa powder, and a sprinkle of sea salt, are a prime example.

These spheres are then formed into bite-sized portions. Alternatively, for a delectable confection that is both straightforward and easy to prepare, roast apple slices with honey and cinnamon. Always opt for unadulterated, whole products to maximize their nutritional value.

CHAPTER EIGHT

Recipes For Special Occasions

Gluten-Free Holiday Recipes

When organizing a gluten-free Christmas feast, it is advisable to consult traditional recipes that are prepared with safe ingredients. Start with a roasted turkey or ham, ensuring that all seasonings and glazes are gluten-free. Serve with a gluten-free stuffing that is made from sautéed vegetables, gluten-free bread, and gluten-free stock.

Accompany the primary course with roasted vegetables, gluten-free gravy, and mashed potatoes. A variety of dessert options are available, including gluten-free pumpkin pie or flourless chocolate cake, to ensure that the meal is enjoyed by all.

Cakes For Birthdays And Celebrations

It may be straightforward and delectable to prepare gluten-free birthday cakes. Substitute a gluten-free flour mix directly into your preferred cake recipe. Store-bought gluten-free flour mixtures, almond flour, and coconut flour are all popular alternatives. Ensure that all other ingredients, such as baking powder and flavorings, are gluten-free. Decorate with gluten-free frosting, colored fruits, or gluten-free sprinkling. Regardless of dietary restrictions, anyone can appreciate a traditional vanilla cake or a rich, delectable chocolate.

Festive Gluten-Free Appetizers

Festive gluten-free refreshments may establish the atmosphere for a pleasurable event. Prepare fresh vegetable crudités with gluten-free dressings or hummus. To prepare gluten-free bruschetta, top gluten-free baguettes with fresh tomatoes, basil, and olive oil. Bacon-wrapped dates or tiny quiches with a gluten-free crust are additional alternatives. These appetizers are not only delectable, but they also cater to individuals who are gluten intolerant without sacrificing flavor.

Main Courses For Special Occasions

Prepare main dishes that are either inherently gluten-free or easily adaptable for special occasions. An elegant centerpiece can be achieved by seasoning a beef tenderloin or rack of lamb with herbs and spices. Combine it with gluten-free side dishes, including steamed asparagus, quinoa salad, or roasted potatoes. Guarantee that any marinades or sauces employed are gluten-free. A stuffing acorn squash with quinoa, cranberries, and pistachios is a vegetarian alternative.

It is imperative to engage in open communication and meticulous planning when hosting a gluten-free celebration. To prevent cross-contamination, it is important to inform visitors about the gluten-free cuisine. Separate culinary areas and equipment should be employed to prepare gluten-free recipes.

Ensure that all gluten-free goods are plainly labeled and stored separately from those that contain gluten.

Guarantee that the munchies and beverages are devoid of gluten. An inclusive and enjoyable experience for all visitors can be achieved by adhering to these procedures.

CHAPTER NINE

Seven Days Meal Plan, Recipes And Detailed Preparatory Guidelines For Celiac Disease

THE FIRST DAY

Breakfast: Banana pancakes that are devoid of gluten.

COMPONENTS:

• Incorporate 1 cup of gluten-free all-purpose flour.

• One tablespoon of sugar

• One teaspoon of baking powder.

• 1/2 teaspoon of baking soda.

• Add 1/4 teaspoon of salt.

• One cup of buttermilk.

• A single, very large egg.

• 2 tablespoons of clarified butter.

• Mash one mature banana.

• One teaspoon of vanilla extract.

PREPARATION:

1. Combine the flour, sugar, baking powder, baking soda, and salt in a sizable basin.

2. Combine the buttermilk, egg, softened butter, banana, and vanilla in a separate dish.

3. Add the liquid ingredients to the dry ingredients and stir until they are combined.

4. Gently apply butter or oil to a nonstick pan that has been heated over medium heat.

5. Pour 1/4 cup of batter onto the skillet for each crepe. Cook until bubbles appear on the surface,

then flip and continue cooking until golden brown.

6. Accompany with fresh produce or maple nectar.

Lunch: Quinoa salad with avocado and legumes.

COMPONENTS:

• One cup of rinsed quinoa

• Two glasses of water.

• 1 can (15 oz) of chickpeas that have been drained and rinsed.

• Cut one avocado into small pieces.

• Cut cherry tomatoes in half and serve one cup.

• Finely mince 1/4 cup of red onion.

• Finely chop 1/4 cup of fresh cilantro.

• The juice of one lime.

• Incorporate 2 tablespoons of olive oil.

• Season with salt and pepper to suit.

PREPARATION:

1. Heat the water and quinoa in a medium saucepan until they reach a simmer. Reduce the heat to a simmer, cover, and cook for 15 minutes or until the water has been absorbed.

2. Combine cooked quinoa, legumes, avocado, cherry tomatoes, red onion, and cilantro in a sizable mixing basin.

3. Combine olive oil, lime juice, salt, and pepper in a small basin.

4. Combine the salad with the vinaigrette by tossing it.

5. Serve at either ambient temperature or refrigerated.

Dinner: Salmon that has been baked with citrus and herbs.

COMPONENTS:

• Four salmon fillets.

• Incorporate 2 tablespoons of olive oil.

• Finely chop two cloves of garlic.

• One lemon juice and rind.

• One tablespoon of dried basil.

• One teaspoon of powdered oregano.

• Season with salt and pepper to suit.

PREPARATION:

1. Preheat the oven to 375° Fahrenheit (190° Celsius).

2. Combine the olive oil, garlic, lemon juice, zest, basil, oregano, salt, and pepper in a small mixing basin.

3. Arrange the salmon fillets on a baking sheet that has been lined with parchment paper.

4. Apply the lemon-herb mixture to the salmon fillets by brushing them.

5. Bake the salmon for 15-20 minutes, or until it is thoroughly cooked and easily flaked with a fork.

6. Accompany with a side salad or sautéed vegetables.

Snack: Apple slices with almond butter.

COMPONENTS:

• One apple, divided.

• 2 tablespoons of almond butter.

PREPARATION:

1. Cut the apple into segments.

2. Accompany with almond butter for dipping.

Juice: Orange-Carrot Juice

COMPONENTS:

• Four large carrots that have been peeled.

• Two oranges that have been skinned.

• One inch of peeled ginger

PREPARATION:

1. Utilize a juicer to extract the liquid from the carrots, citrus, and ginger.

2. Stir the juice and serve immediately.

THE SECOND DAY

COMPONENTS:

• One cup of Greek yogurt.

• Incorporate 1/2 cup of gluten-free granola.

• Combine 1/2 cup of assorted fruit (strawberries, raspberries, and blueberries).

• Optional: Incorporate 1 tablespoon of honey.

PREPARATION:

1. Transfer the Greek yogurt to a basin by spooning it.

2. Garnish with a mixture of assorted berries and gluten-free granola.

3. If desired, drizzle with honey.

COMPONENTS:

- One cup of rinsed legumes

- One onion, finely diced.

- Chop two carrots.

- Cut two stalks of celery into small pieces.

- Three bulbs of garlic should be minced.

- One can (14.5 oz) of diced tomatoes.

- Six cups of vegetable bouillon.

- Add 1 teaspoon of dried thyme.

- One teaspoon of dried rosemary.

- Season with salt and pepper to suit.

PREPARATION:

1. Sauté the onion, carrots, and celery in a large saucepan until they are tender.

2. Add the garlic and continue to simmer for an additional minute.

3. Combine the legumes, diced tomatoes, vegetable broth, thyme, rosemary, salt, and pepper.

4. Bring the mixture to a boil, then reduce the heat and allow it to simmer for 30 minutes, or until the lentils are fully cooked.

5. Present the dish steaming, accompanied by gluten-free crostini.

COMPONENTS:

• Discard the seeds and crowns of four bell peppers.

• One pound of ground beef or poultry.

• One cup of cooked gluten-free rice.

• 1 can (15 oz) of black beans that have been strained and rinsed.

• One cup of maize seeds.

• One cup of salsa.

• Utilize one teaspoon of cardamom.

• Add one (1) teaspoon of paprika.

• Season with salt and pepper to suit.

• Shredded cheese, 1 cup, is an optional addition.

PREPARATION:

1. Preheat the oven to 375° Fahrenheit (190° Celsius).

2. Brown the minced beef in a large pan. Remove any surplus fat.

3. Combine the cooked rice, black beans, maize, salsa, cumin, paprika, salt, and pepper.

4. Place the bell peppers in a roasting dish and fill them with the meat mixture.

5. If cheese is employed, distribute it over the filled chiles.

6. Bake the dish for thirty minutes with the foil covering it. Bake for an additional 10 minutes after removing the foil.

7. Serve the dish at a high temperature.

COMPONENTS:

• Peel and mince two large carrots into spears.

• Incorporate 1/2 cup of humus.

PREPARATION:

1. Slice carrots into pieces.

2. Accompany with tahini for dipping.

COMPONENTS:

• Two cups of spinach.

• One cucumber.

• Two pears that are still green.

• One lemon that has been sliced.

• One inch of peeled ginger

PREPARATION:

1. Utilize a juicer to extract the juice from the cucumber, green fruits, lemon, and ginger.

2. Stir the juice and serve immediately.

THIRD DAY

Breakfast: Mango Chia Seed Pudding

COMPONENTS:

• Chia seeds, 1/4 cup.

• Incorporate 1 cup of almond milk (or another plant-based milk).

• One tablespoon of maple syrup.

• Incorporate 1/2 teaspoon of vanilla essence.

• Chop one mature mango into small pieces.

PREPARATION:

1. Combine the almond milk, maple syrup, vanilla extract, and chia seeds in a basin.

2. Stir the mixture thoroughly to prevent clumping, and then refrigerate it overnight.

3. In the morning, combine the pudding and add sliced mango as a garnish.

4. Serve chilled.

Lunch: Chicken and Avocado Lettuce Wraps

COMPONENTS:

• Shred one pound of cooked chicken breast.

• One avocado, diced.

• Cherry tomatoes, halved (1/2 cup).

• Finely mince 1/4 cup of red onion.

• One tablespoon of lime juice.

• Divide a single head of romaine or iceberg lettuce into individual leaves.

• Season with salt and pepper to suit.

PREPARATION:

1. Combine the shredded chicken, avocado, cherry tomatoes, red onion, lime juice, salt, and pepper in a basin.

2. Thoroughly combine to achieve a uniform mixture.

3. Spoon the mixture onto the lettuce leaves.

4. Serve immediately.

Dinner: Quinoa topped with grilled prawn skewers.

COMPONENTS:

• One-pound shrimp were peeled and deveined.

• Incorporate 2 tablespoons of olive oil.

• Finely chop two cloves of garlic.

• The juice of one lemon.

• Add one (1) teaspoon of paprika.

• Season with salt and pepper to suit.

• One cup of rinsed quinoa

• Two glasses of water.

PREPARATION:

1. Prepare the barbecue for medium-high heat.

2. Combine olive oil, garlic, lemon juice, paprika, salt, and pepper in a basin.

3. Allow the shrimp to marinate for 15 minutes.

4. Thread the shrimp onto skewers and grill for 2-3 minutes on each side, or until they are fully cooked.

5. In the meantime, bring the quinoa and water to a simmer in a medium saucepan. Reduce the heat to a simmer, cover, and cook for 15 minutes or until the water has been absorbed.

6. Accompany the shrimp skewers with the quinoa that has been prepared.

Snack: Rice cakes topped with banana and peanut butter.

COMPONENTS:

• Two rice cakes.

• Two teaspoons of peanut butter.

• One banana, diced.

PREPARATION:

1. Apply peanut butter to each rice cake.

2. Add banana segments on top.

3. Serve immediately.

Pineapple and cucumber juice

COMPONENTS:

• Cut and peel half of the pineapple.

• One cucumber.

• Peel one-half of a lemon.

PREPARATION:

1. Utilize a centrifuge to extract the liquid from the pineapple, cucumber, and lemon.

2. Stir the juice and serve immediately.

THE FOURTH DAY

COMPONENTS:

• One banana that has been chilled.

• Incorporate 1/2 cup of thawed fruit.

• Incorporate 1/2 cup of almond milk.

• 1 tablespoon of chia seeds

• Incorporate 1/4 cup of gluten-free granola.

PREPARATION:

1. Combine the frozen banana, frozen berries, almond milk, and chia seeds in a blender until the mixture is smooth.

2. Transfer the mixture to a basin and top it off with gluten-free granola.

3. Serve immediately.

COMPONENTS:

• Cut two substantial tomatoes into slices.

• Cut one fresh mozzarella ball into slices.

• One-quarter cup of fresh basil leaves.

• Incorporate 2 teaspoons of balsamic vinegar.

• Incorporate 2 tablespoons of olive oil.

• Season with salt and pepper to suit.

PREPARATION:

1. Arrange the tomato and mozzarella slices on a platter in alternating order.

2. Insert the basil leaves between the segments.

3. Drizzle with olive oil and balsamic vinegar.

4. Season with salt and pepper.

5. Serve immediately.

Dinner: Chicken Parmesan that is devoid of gluten.

COMPONENTS:

• Two chicken breasts that are boneless and skinless.

• Incorporate 1/2 cup of gluten-free breadcrumbs.

• Incorporate 1/4 cup of grated Parmesan cheese.

• One teaspoon of powdered oregano.

• One egg that has been pounded.

• One cup of gluten-free marinara sauce.

• One cup of grated mozzarella cheese.

PREPARATION:

1. Preheat the oven to 375° Fahrenheit (190° Celsius).

2. In a combining basin, combine the oregano, Parmesan cheese, and gluten-free breadcrumbs.

3. Dip the chicken breasts into the beaten egg, then coat them with the breadcrumb mixture.

4. Arrange the chicken breasts that have been marinated on a baking sheet that has been lined with parchment paper.

5. Bake for 20 minutes, then remove from the oven and distribute marinara sauce on each slice.

6. Sprinkle with grated mozzarella and continue baking for an additional 10 minutes, or until the cheese is softened and steaming.

7. Serve the dish fresh, accompanied by a side of gluten-free pasta or salad.

Snack: Cream cheese-covered celery stalks.

COMPONENTS:

• Slice three celery stalks into pieces.

• One-fourth cup of cream cheese.

PREPARATION:

1. Apply cream cheese to each celery stalk.

2. Serve immediately.

Beetroot-apple juice

COMPONENTS:

• Cut and peel two beets.

• Two apples that have been cored and sliced.

• One inch of peeled ginger

PREPARATION:

1. Utilize a centrifuge to extract the liquid from the beets, apples, and ginger.

2. Stir the juice and serve immediately.

DAY FIVE

Breakfast: An omelet topped with feta and vegetables.

COMPONENTS:

• Three eggs

• Add 1/4 cup of almond milk or milk.

• Finely chop one cup of fresh spinach.

• 1/4 cup of shredded feta cheese.

• Season with salt and pepper to suit.

• One tablespoon of olive oil

PREPARATION:

1. In a combining dish, whisk the eggs and milk until they are thoroughly combined. Add salt and pepper to taste.

2. Heat the olive oil in a nonstick skillet over medium heat.

3. Add the spinach and simmer until it is wilted.

4. Pour the egg mixture into the skillet and heat until it begins to set.

5. Sprinkle feta cheese over one-half of the omelet.

6. Fold the omelette in half and continue cooking for an additional 1-2 minutes, or until the eggs are thoroughly set.

7. Serve the dish at a high temperature.

COMPONENTS:

• One gluten-free tortilla.

• Four slices of poultry breast.

• Slice one-half of an avocado.

• 1/4 cup of shredded lettuce.

• Add 2 tablespoons of mayonnaise.

• Season with salt and pepper to suit.

PREPARATION:

1. Apply the mayonnaise to the gluten-free tortillas.

2. Arrange turkey slices, avocado, and shredded lettuce on top.

3. Season with salt and pepper.

4. Fold the tortilla in half and roll it up.

5. Serve immediately.

COMPONENTS:

• Cut four medium zucchinis in half lengthwise and remove the seeds.

• One pound of ground beef or poultry

• Chop half of an onion.

• Finely chop two cloves of garlic.

• One cup of gluten-free marinara sauce

• Incorporate 1/2 cup of grated Parmesan cheese.

• One cup of grated mozzarella cheese

• Season with salt and pepper to suit.

PREPARATION:

1. Preheat the oven to 375° Fahrenheit (190° Celsius).

2. Brown the minced beef in a large pan. Sauté the garlic and onion until they are tender.

3. Substitute the marinara sauce and continue to simmer for an additional five minutes.

4. Spoon the meat mixture into the zucchinis that have been hollowed out.

5. Garnish with shredded mozzarella and grated Parmesan.

6. Arrange the zucchini boats on a baking sheet and bake for 25-30 minutes, or until the cheese has melted and bubbled and the zucchini is tender.

7. Serve the dish at a high temperature.

COMPONENTS:

• 1/4 cup of a variety of nuts, including pistachios, almonds, and walnuts.

PREPARATION:

1. As a quick and nutritious refreshment, offer a small bowl of assorted nuts.

COMPONENTS:

• Two cups of kale

• Cut and peel half of the pineapple.

• One green apple.

• Peel one-half of a lemon.

PREPARATION:

1. Utilize a juicer to extract the juice from the kale, pineapple, green apple, and lemon.

2. Stir the juice and serve immediately.

SIXTH DAY

Breakfast: Blueberry Oatmeal Prepared Overnight

COMPONENTS:

• Incorporate 1/2 cup of gluten-free cereals.

• Incorporate 1 cup of almond milk (or another plant-based milk).

• 1 tablespoon of chia seeds

• One tablespoon of maple syrup

• One-half cup of blueberries.

PREPARATION:

1. Combine the cereals, almond milk, chia seeds, and maple syrup in a container or dish.

2. Mix thoroughly and refrigerate overnight.

3. Add fresh blueberries to the dish in the morning.

4. Serve chilled.

Lunch: Grilled chicken with a Greek salad.

COMPONENTS:

• Two bowls of assorted greens.

• Cut one-half of a cucumber into thin slices.

• Cherry tomatoes, halved (1/2 cup).

• Thinly slice 1/4 of a red onion.

• Incorporate 1/4 cup of Kalamata olives.

• 1/4 cup of shredded feta cheese.

• One broiled chicken breast, sliced.

• Incorporate 2 tablespoons of olive oil.

• One tablespoon of red wine vinegar.

• Season with salt and pepper to suit.

PREPARATION:

1. Combine the greens, cucumber, cherry tomatoes, red onion, olives, and feta cheese in a sizable mixing basin.

2. Add diced seared chicken breast to the top.

3. Combine the olive oil, red wine vinegar, salt, and pepper in a small basin.

4. Apply the vinaigrette to the salad and combine.

5. Serve immediately.

COMPONENTS:

• Four halibut fillets.

• Incorporate 2 tablespoons of olive oil.

• Finely chop two cloves of garlic.

• Add 1 teaspoon of dried thyme.

• 1 teaspoon of dried parsley.

• The juice of one lemon.

• Season with salt and pepper to suit.

PREPARATION:

1. Preheat the oven to 375° Fahrenheit (190° Celsius).

2. Combine olive oil, garlic, thyme, parsley, lemon juice, salt, and pepper in a small basin.

3. Arrange the fish fillets on a baking pan that has been lined with parchment paper.

4. Apply the garlic-herb mixture to the salmon fillets by brushing them.

5. Bake the fish for 15-20 minutes, or until it is thoroughly cooked and easily flaked with a utensil.

6. Accompany with a steamed vegetable or salad.

Snack: Cheese and Crackers that is gluten-free

COMPONENTS:

• A total of ten gluten-free wafers.

• 1/4 cup of cubed cheese, such as gouda or cheddar.

PREPARATION:

1. Accompany slices of cheese with gluten-free crackers.

Watermelon-mint juice

COMPONENTS:

• Two tablespoons of diced watermelon

• Half of a cucumber.

• Fresh mint leaves, 1/4 cup.

PREPARATION:

1. Utilize a juicer to extract the liquid from the cucumber, watermelon, and mint sprigs.

2. Stir the juice and serve immediately.

SEVENTH DAY

COMPONENTS:

• Two slices of gluten-free bread.

• One mature avocado.

• One tablespoon of lemon juice

• Season with salt and pepper to suit.

• Radish segments, cherry tomatoes, and poached eggs are among the optional garnishes.

PREPARATION:

1. Toast the gluten-free baguette slices.

2. Mash the avocado in a basin and add the lemon juice, salt, and pepper.

3. Apply the pureed avocado to the toasted bread.

4. Optional garnishes may be incorporated if desired.

5. Serve immediately.

Lunch: Tuna salad lettuce rolls.

COMPONENTS:

• One drained can of tuna (5 ounces)

• Utilize 1/4 cup of mayonnaise.

• One tablespoon of Dijon mustard.

• 1/4 cup of celery that has been sliced

• Finely chop 1/4 cup of red onion.

• Season with salt and pepper to suit.

• Divide a single head of romaine or iceberg lettuce into individual leaves.

PREPARATION:

1. Combine the tuna, celery, red onion, Dijon mustard, mayonnaise, and salt and pepper in a basin.

2. Thoroughly combine to achieve a uniform mixture.

3. Spoon tuna salad onto lettuce leaves.

4. Serve immediately.

Dinner: Spaghetti and meatballs that are gluten-free

COMPONENTS:

• One box of gluten-free spaghetti.

• One pound of ground beef or poultry.

• Utilize 1/4 cup of gluten-free breadcrumbs.

• Incorporate 1/4 cup of grated Parmesan cheese.

• One egg that has been pounded.

• One teaspoon of powdered oregano.

• One tablespoon of dried basil.

• Season with salt and pepper to suit.

• Utilize two cups of gluten-free marinara sauce.

PREPARATION:

1. Prepare the gluten-free linguine by the cooking instructions provided on the packaging.

2. In a basin, combine the minced beef, gluten-free breadcrumbs, Parmesan cheese, beaten egg, oregano, basil, salt, and pepper.

3. Form the mixture into meatballs and arrange them on a baking sheet that has been lined with parchment paper.

4. Bake the meatballs at 375°F (190°C) for 20 minutes or until they are completely cooked.

5. Heat the marinara sauce in a sizable saucepan. Boil the meatballs that have been prepared for 10 minutes.

6. Accompany the cooked pasta with the meatballs and sauce.

7. If desired, add a sprinkle of Parmesan cheese.

Snack: A mélange of fresh produce.

COMPONENTS:

• One cup of cut strawberries.

• One cup of blackberries.

• One cup of chopped pineapple.

• One diced kiwi.

PREPARATION:

1. Combine the kiwi, pineapple, blueberries, and strawberries in a basin.

2. Gently integrate by mixing.

3. Serve immediately.

Apple, carrot, and ginger juice

COMPONENTS:

• Two apples that have been cored and sliced.

• Three large carrots, peeled

• One inch of peeled ginger

PREPARATION:

1. Utilize a juicer to extract the liquid from the fruits, carrots, and ginger.

2. Stir the juice and serve immediately.

CHAPTER TEN

Seven Dessert Recipes And Guidelines For Celiac Disease

Celiac disease necessitates a strict gluten-free diet; however, this does not entail the abandonment of exquisite delights. The following are seven delectable recipes that are suitable for individuals with celiac disease, as well as recommendations for safe preparation.

1. CHOCOLATE CAKE WITHOUT FLOUR

COMPONENTS:

• One cup of unsalted butter.

• Eight ounces. diced semisweet chocolate.

• 1 1/4 cups of refined sugar.

• Six large eggs.

• One cup of cocoa powder.

STEPS:

1. Preheat the oven to 350° Fahrenheit (175° Celsius). Cover the bottom of a 9-inch springform pan with parchment paper and grease it.

2. In a saucepan over low heat, melt the butter and chocolate by stirring until the mixture is homogeneous.

3. Remove from the flame, add the sugar, and mix thoroughly.

4. Whisk the eggs until they are fully incorporated, adding them one at a time.

5. Whisk the cocoa powder into the mixture until it is fully incorporated.

6. Transfer the mixture to the prepared pan and bake for 25–30 minutes.

7. Allow the dish to settle in the pan before removing it. Before serving, sprinkle with cocoa powder or powdered sugar.

2. COOKIES MADE WITH ALMOND FLOUR

COMPONENTS:

• Two cups of almond flour.

• Incorporate 1/2 cup of coconut sugar.

• Melt 1/4 cup of coconut oil.

• Incorporate 1 teaspoon of vanilla essence.

• A single, very large egg.

• Incorporate 1/2 teaspoon of baking soda.

• Add 1/4 teaspoon of salt.

• 1/2 cup of dark chocolate morsels (gluten-free).

STEPS:

1. Preheat the oven to 350° Fahrenheit (175° Celsius). Line a baking sheet with parchment paper.

2. Combine almond flour, coconut sugar, baking soda, and salt in a sizable basin.

3. In an additional container, combine vanilla essence, egg, and coconut oil.

4. Combine the moist and dry ingredients and stir until they are fully incorporated.

5. Incorporate the chocolate morsels.

6. Place tablespoon-sized spheres onto the baking sheet and gently press them down.

7. Bake for 10-12 minutes, or until the edges are a rich golden brown.

8. Allow the baked goods to settle on the baking pan for five minutes before transferring them to a wire rack.

COMPONENTS:

• For the crust:

Utilize one cup of gluten-free all-purpose flour.

Utilize 1/2 cup of softened unsalted butter.

Add 1/4 cup of granulated sugar.

• To fill:

Add 1 1/2 cups of granulated sugar.

Utilize 1/4 cup of gluten-free flour.

There are four very large embryos.

2/3 cup of lemon juice.

STEPS:

1. Preheat the oven to 350° Fahrenheit (175° Celsius). Grease an 8-by-8-inch casserole tin.

2. To prepare the crust, mix flour, butter, and granulated sugar until it is crumbly. Press the mixture into the dish's base.

3. Bake for 20 minutes or until the surface is lightly caramelized.

4. Combine sugar, flour, eggs, and lemon juice to create the filling.

5. Pour the filling over the heated crust and continue baking for an additional 20-25 minutes.

6. Allow the mixture to chill completely before cutting it into bars. Before serving, sprinkle granulated sugar over the dish.

COMPONENTS:

• Four large egg yolks.

• One cup of refined sugar.

• Incorporate 1/2 teaspoon of vanilla essence.

• Incorporate 2 1/2 cups of desiccated shredded coconut.

STEPS:

1. Preheat the oven to 325° Fahrenheit (165° Celsius). Line a baking sheet with parchment paper.

2. In a sizable mixing bowl, whisk the egg whites until they become frothy. Gradually incorporate the sugar and continue to stir until firm peaks are achieved.

3. Gently incorporate the grated coconut and vanilla extract into the mixture.

4. Arrange tablespoon-sized mounds on the baking sheet that has been preheated.

5. Bake for 20-25 minutes, or until the edges are a rich golden brown.

6. Allow the dish to cool on the baking sheet before transferring it to a wire rack.

5. RICE PUDDING

COMPONENTS:

• One cup of uncooked white rice.

• Two glasses of water.

• Four glasses of milk (or a non-dairy alternative)

• Sugar, 3/4 cup.

• Incorporate 1 teaspoon of vanilla essence.

- Incorporate 1/2 teaspoon of powdered cinnamon.

STEPS:

1. Heat water and rice in a medium saucepan until they reach a simmer. Reduce the heat, cover, and allow the mixture to simmer for 20 minutes.

2. Combine the cooked rice, milk, sugar, and vanilla in an additional sizable saucepan. Stir frequently over medium heat until the mixture is viscous and velvety, which should take approximately 20 to 25 minutes.

3. Toss in the cinnamon after removing from the flame.

4. Serve the dish either heated or chilled.

COMPONENTS:

• Utilize one cup of gluten-free peanut butter (refer to the packaging).

• One cup of refined sugar.

• A single, very large egg.

• Add 1 teaspoon of baking soda.

STEPS:

1. Preheat the oven to 350° Fahrenheit (175° Celsius). Line a baking sheet with parchment paper.

2. Combine all of the ingredients in a large combining basin and stir until the mixture is homogeneous.

3. Place spoonfuls of dough onto the baking tray that has been preheated.

4. Utilize a spatula to flatten the mixture to establish a crisscross pattern.

5. Bake for 10–12 minutes or until the edges are firm.

6. Allow the dish to cool on the baking sheet before transferring it to a wire rack.

7. BERRY PARFAIT.

COMPONENTS:

• Incorporate 2 cups of a combination of berries, including raspberries, blueberries, and strawberries.

• Incorporate 2 containers of gluten-free Greek yogurt.

• Utilize 1/4 cup of honey.

• Incorporate 1/4 cup of gluten-free granola.

1. Combine the honey and berries in a medium-sized dish.

2. Arrange the yogurt, berry mélange, and granola in serving glasses.

3. Repeat the layering process, either serving immediately or marinating for a later date.

Baking Guidelines For Gluten-Free Products

1. Thoroughly Examine Product Labels: It is imperative to verify that all constituents are gluten-free by reviewing the product label.

2. When preparing gluten-free, it is important to use separate utensils, mixing basins, and baking trays to prevent cross-contamination.

3. Employ Certified Gluten-Free Products: Ensure that all flours, baking powders, and other baking ingredients are labeled gluten-free.

4. Opt for gluten-free flour, such as almond flour, coconut flour, or certified gluten-free all-purpose flour mixtures.

5. To prevent contamination, it is important to store gluten-free ingredients and baked products in separate locations from those that contain gluten.

6. Thoroughly clean the area before and after preparing gluten-free delights.

By adhering to these recipes and instructions, you will be able to indulge in a variety of treats that are safe, delicious, and suitable for individuals with celiac disease.

CHAPTER ELEVEN

Seven Smoothies Procedural Recipes For Celiac Disease And Guidelines

Celiac disease necessitates stringent adherence to a gluten-free diet, which can frequently be perceived as restrictive. Nevertheless, smoothies are a delectable and adaptable method of incorporating a diverse selection of healthful ingredients into your daily routine. Seven gluten-free smoothie recipes are presented below, each of which is abundant in essential nutrients.

1. GREEN DETOX SMOOTHIE

COMPONENTS:

• One cup of spinach.

• Incorporate 1/2 cup of kale.

• Cut and core one green apple.

• Cut one-half of a cucumber into thin slices.

• One-half of an avocado.

• One cup of coconut water.

• The juice of one lemon.

DIRECTIONS:

1. In a blender, combine avocado, cucumber, apple, kale, and spinach.

2. Incorporate the lemon juice and coconut water.

3. Process the ingredients on high until it's smooth.

4. Pour the beverage into a vessel and consume it immediately.

Instructions: Thoroughly rinse all fresh produce. This smoothie is an excellent detox option due to its high fiber, vitamin, and antioxidant content.

COMPONENTS:

• Combine 1 cup of assorted fruit (strawberries, raspberries, and blueberries).

• One banana.

• Incorporate 1/2 cup of gluten-free Greek yogurt.

• 1 tablespoon of chia seeds

• One cup of almond milk.

DIRECTIONS:

1. In a blender, combine the chia seeds, Greek yogurt, banana, and cherries.

2. Incorporate the almond milk.

3. Blend until the mixture is velvety and smooth.

4. Serve immediately.

Antioxidants and vitamin C are abundant in mixed berries. Greek yogurt contains probiotics that are beneficial for digestive health, making it particularly beneficial for individuals with celiac disease.

3. SMOOTHIE WITH PINEAPPLE AND TROPICAL MANGO

COMPONENTS:

• One cup of mango segments, either fresh or chilled.

• One cup of pineapple segments, either fresh or chilled.

• Incorporate 1/2 cup of orange juice.

• Incorporate 1/2 cup of coconut milk.

• One tablespoon of flaxseeds.

DIRECTIONS:

1. Combine the mango, pineapple, citrus juice, and coconut milk in a blender.

2. Incorporate flaxseeds.

3. Blend until the mixture is frothy and smooth.

4. Take pleasure in the present moment.

Guideline: This smoothie is rich in vitamin C and has a delectable tropical flavor. Guarantee that the orange juice is entirely juice and does not contain any gluten-containing additives.

4. SMOOTHIE WITH BANANAS AND PEANUT BUTTER

COMPONENTS:

• Two avocados.

• Before utilizing two tablespoons of peanut butter, verify that it is gluten-free.

• Utilize one cup of gluten-free oat milk.

• One tablespoon of honey.

• 1/4 teaspoon of cinnamon.

DIRECTIONS:

1. Combine the bananas, peanut butter, oat milk, honey, and cinnamon in the Vitamix.

2. Blend until the mixture is velvety and smooth.

3. Pour the beverage into a glass and savor it.

Guideline: Bananas and peanut butter are a conventional combination that is rich in protein, healthful lipids, and potassium. Always verify that your oat milk is gluten-free, as oats can frequently be cross-contaminated with gluten.

COMPONENTS:

• One avocado.

• One cup of coconut milk.

• One tablespoon of maple syrup.

• Incorporate 1/2 teaspoon of vanilla essence.

• Add 1/2 cup of ice crystals.

DIRECTIONS:

1. Transfer the avocado to a processor.

2. Combine the ice crystals, maple syrup, vanilla essence, and coconut milk.

3. Blend until the mixture is velvety and smooth.

4. Serve chilled.

Guideline: This smoothie is rich in healthful lipids and has a luxuriant, creamy texture. Without the addition of refined sugar, maple syrup offers a subtle sweetness.

6. PROTEIN POWER SMOOTHIE

COMPONENTS:

• One spoonful of gluten-free protein powder.

• One banana.

• One cup of almond milk.

• One tablespoon of almond butter.

• Incorporate 1/2 teaspoon of chocolate powder.

DIRECTIONS:

1. Combine protein powder, banana, almond milk, almond butter, and chocolate powder in a blender.

2. Blend the mixture until it is perfectly homogeneous.

3. Pour the beverage into a glass and savor it.

Guideline: This smoothie is an excellent choice for post-workout recovery or as a meal replacement. Ensure that your protein powder is certified gluten-free to prevent contamination.

7. SMOOTHIE MADE WITH FRESH WATERMELON AND MINT

COMPONENTS:

• Two cups of cubed cantaloupe.

• 1/2 cup of hulled strawberries.

• The juice of one lime.

• A few fresh mint sprigs.

• Add 1/2 cup of ice crystals.

DIRECTIONS:

1. Combine the cantaloupe, strawberries, lime juice, and mint sprigs in a blender.

2. Incorporate ice crystals.

3. Blend until the mixture is homogeneous and invigorating.

4. Serve immediately.

Guideline: This smoothie is particularly hydrating and well-suited for humid weather. Mint enhances the refreshing flavor of watermelon, which is low in calories and high in vitamins A and C.

In conclusion, while adhering to a gluten-free diet that is suitable for celiac disease, these seven smoothies offer a diverse array of nutrients and flavors. By incorporating these smoothies into your daily regimen, you can ensure that your health and well-being are benefited by a diverse and nutritious diet. Label all packaged ingredients as gluten-free to prevent cross-contamination. These smoothie recipes are both safe and delicious, so you can enjoy your voyage to improved health.

CHAPTER TWELVE

Strategies For Long-Term Gluten-Free Living

Maintaining a well-stocked kitchen with gluten-free essentials, including gluten-free pasta, quinoa, and rice, is crucial for maintaining a gluten-free lifestyle over an extended period. It is imperative to consistently review food labels to prevent the consumption of seasonings and sauces that contain gluten.

Batch-cook and preserve dishes to facilitate the availability of gluten-free options. Learn how to make gluten-free bread and desserts so that you can savor your beloved dishes. To enhance your diet and maintain interest in your dishes, consider incorporating gluten-free flours such as almond, coconut, and rice flour.

Maintaining A Positive And Motivated State Of Mind

Celebrate small victories, such as learning a new gluten-free recipe or uncovering a new gluten-free restaurant, to maintain a positive attitude and stay motivated while adhering to a gluten-free diet. Maintain a journal to track your progress and assess the extent to which you are experiencing physical and psychological enhancements. Assemble a support system of acquaintances and family members who comprehend your nutritional requirements. Consider the benefits of a gluten-free lifestyle, including improved health and well-being, rather than worrying about what you are giving up.

Locating Community And Support

It is imperative to establish a support system and community to sustain a gluten-free diet. Participate in local or online celiac disease support groups to exchange recipes, suggestions, and personal experiences. Engage in gluten-free activities, such as food festivals or culinary courses, to connect with individuals who understand your challenges. Follow gluten-free bloggers and influencers to receive daily inspiration and advice. Engage with these communities consistently to experience a sense of empowerment and lessen the sense of isolation during your gluten-free journey.

Dining Out And Traveling Gluten-Free

Precise preparation is required for gluten-free dining and travel. Locate gluten-free restaurants in your vicinity and assess them from other gluten-free diners. Carry gluten-free treats, including dried fruit and almonds, to alleviate hunger when there are few alternatives. Inform the staff of your dietary restrictions and specifically inquire about the preparation of the food when dining out. Staying in accommodations that include a kitchen allows you to prepare a portion of your meals gluten-free.

Resources And Continuing Education

It is imperative to maintain one's understanding of celiac disease and gluten-free lifestyles through the use of resources and continuing education. For the most up-to-date information, recipes, and ideas regarding celiac disease, subscribe to newsletters and magazines.

Participate in conferences and seminars on celiac disease to gain knowledge from professionals and establish connections with others in the community. Utilize reputable gluten-free websites and applications to locate safe restaurants and products. Ensure that you have a collection of gluten-free cookbooks to expand your culinary options and enhance the enjoyment of your diet.

Conclusion

In summary, the "Celiac Disease Diet Cookbook" is an indispensable resource for individuals who are facing the challenges of gluten-free living as a result of celiac disease. This cookbook not only offers a diverse selection of nutritious, safe, and delectable dishes, but it also educates readers on the importance of avoiding gluten and the potential health risks associated with cross-contamination. It offers comprehensive guidance on the selection of food, meal preparation, and cooking techniques, enabling individuals to prepare delicious and nutritious meals.

Additionally, the cookbook emphasizes the importance of a well-balanced diet, which guarantees that celiac disease patients do not miss out on essential vitamins and minerals that are frequently found in gluten-containing products. Readers may sustain a diet that is both diverse and enjoyable by incorporating a variety of cereals, fruits, vegetables, and proteins. Practical insights and encouragement are provided by testimonials and recommendations from celiac disease patients, which foster a supportive community among readers.

Lastly, the "Celiac Disease Diet Cookbook" is not merely a compilation of recipes; it is a source of inspiration and an instructional aid for individuals who are committed to a gluten-free lifestyle. It illustrates the potential of maintaining a healthy lifestyle and enjoying food with joy, despite the challenges posed by celiac disease.

THE END